In My Shoes

In My Shoes

✦

A Journey to Living Well with Multiple Sclerosis

Mary Monaghan Sypawka

iUniverse, Inc.
New York Lincoln Shanghai

In My Shoes
A Journey to Living Well with Multiple Sclerosis

iUniverse books may be ordered through booksellers or by contacting:

iUniverse
2021 Pine Lake Road, Suite 100
Lincoln, NE 68512
www.iuniverse.com
1-800-Authors (1-800-288-4677)

Because of the dynamic nature of the Internet, any Web addresses or links contained in this book may have changed since publication and may no longer be valid.

The views expressed in this work are solely those of the author and do not necessarily reflect the views of the publisher, and the publisher hereby disclaims any responsibility for them.

ISBN: 978-0-595-44446-5 (pbk)
ISBN: 978-0-595-88772-9 (ebk)

Printed in the United States of America

To my family and friends, especially Steve, Mom, and Dad

Words I try to live by:

"We have one solid source of happiness in all our journeying—we can keep our hearts fixed on God."

—Catherine McAuley

"Be who you are and say what you feel, because those who mind don't matter and those who matter don't mind."

—Dr. Seuss

"I am only one; but still I am one. I cannot do everything, but still I can do something. I will not refuse to do the something I can do."

—Helen Keller

"Hope is the feeling you have that the feeling you have isn't permanent."

—Jean Kerr

"The only way to have a friend is to be one."

—Ralph Waldo Emerson

Contents

Foreword

This book began as a journal, reminiscent of one of those diaries I had as a kid. I just loved those little books, with their tiny keys. I remember I had a little red diary in which I wrote about my first crushes, details of conversations with my girlfriends, and complaints about getting scolded in school for talking too much. I could write to my heart's content and then lock the diary, in hopes that I was preventing my four older brothers and everyone else from unlocking the book and finding out my secrets.

Like the contents of my diary, I kept all my MS secrets locked up, for many reasons. My doctor suggested that I use a journal as a way to release those pent-up secrets. I was astonished to find out that journaling was quite therapeutic. The writing helped me to express my thoughts and feelings, without the pressure of a clock ticking off the forty-five minutes of a therapy session or the difficulty I sometimes had with saying some things out loud to another person.

After I figured out that I actually enjoyed writing, my vision soon became to write a book that could be helpful, amusing or educational to others, who, like me, have multiple sclerosis. And, because my husband and I are geeks, we decided to take it a step further and parlay the writing effort into a Web site, with the same goal of helping people with multiple sclerosis or their friends and families through my personal experiences.

Thus, *In My Shoes*, and our Web site, www.livewellwithms.com, were born. The effort has been, and continues to be, quite a learning experience. It is not only cathartic, but my way of educating people about my real-bottom line, no-holds-barred-life experiences with multiple sclerosis. I initially planned on using a pen name, but decided against it when I recognized that a pen name defeated my goal of communicating honestly. I have chosen to use fictitious names throughout my writing in order to protect my family and friends' privacy.

Throughout the course of my illness, I found that the majority of reading material relating to MS was often quite clinical, over my head or just plain depressing. I had so many unanswered questions like: What symptoms do other people with MS experience? How does the illness progress? How do they feel about having MS? How do other people treat them? How do they deal with everyday-life MS challenges?

After more than a decade of living with MS, I feel like a veteran! I hope that by sharing some of my pitfalls and coping mechanisms, it may provide other persons with MS and their families answers to some of their questions and suggestions for living well with multiple sclerosis.

1

My Black Suede Shoes

Ever since I was a little girl, I have always loved shoes. My friends and I used to play dress-up, and it always included a pair of someone's old high heels. I remember my white, patent-leather Easter shoes. I had black, patent-leather Mary Janes, too. I remember the Christmas when Santa delivered go-go boots for me. Summer footwear included flip-flops and sneakers—and remember those wooden sandals that were supposed to feel good on your feet but didn't? When I was in grade school, saddle shoes and penny loafers were absolutely a necessity. There was the Earth-shoe phase; they were the most comfortable and ugliest shoes I have ever owned. Finally, who can forget desert boots?

I remember that the best part of going back to school after the summer was that trip to the shoe store. I loved the smell of leather—and still do. It reminds me of September, crisp apples, spiced wafers, and falling leaves.

Somewhere around the seventh grade came the realization that I was short. That realization began my love affair with platform shoes and clogs, with me hoping that I would get those inches that made me more than five feet tall. In high school, my attempt to be cool wearing a plain, green uniform was to have colorful, sparkly socks and neat shoes. Upon my entry into the business world, I was thrilled that I could buy and wear my own high heels. I had every imaginable color, height, and style, and panty hose and leggings to match all of them.

And when I started tripping over my own feet and stumbled more than I walked, I resigned myself to flats—but it's impossible to be stylish or tall in flats.

When I was diagnosed with multiple sclerosis, I found that there were many changes that I would have to accept in my life. Some of the changes

1

were more acceptable than others. It may seem silly to some people, but for me, one of the biggest personal indignities of having multiple sclerosis is not being able to wear shoes that I really like. When a special occasion comes along, and I find that perfect dress, it is quite depressing that I can't wear a great pair of satin pumps, bejeweled sandals or sequined heels to match the outfit.

After I resigned myself to wearing sensible shoes, it took me a long time to give away my heels. Deep down inside, I really thought that I would wear them again. But, eventually, I finally donated them to a worthy cause—except for one pair. I just couldn't stand to part with them.

A few years ago, long before Ellen made Life Lists fashionable, I created a list of things that I wanted to accomplish. The list contained items such as "Be nicer to my husband," "Spend more time with my friends," "Be more religious," "Be more religious about taking my MS medicines," and last, but not least, "WEAR HEELS AGAIN!" Remember that one pair that I didn't give away? Those, I had decided, would be the first ones that I would wear. They are beautiful, black suede, three-inch high-heel pumps.

I am a goal-oriented person. Because of that, I have made changes in my lifestyle that will help me reach my goal. I like to think that I am keeping myself ready for that cure. I do not want to regress to a point where a new drug discovery won't help me.

Whether you have multiple sclerosis, are an MS caregiver or family member, have another chronic illness, or just like to read, I invite you to journey with me and find out what it's like to be in my shoes. Maybe you will learn something new, or maybe you will be able to better understand what someone you love is going through. Much of my story relates not only to MS, but to chronic illness in general.

Now, then—let's start that journey ...

2

What is MS and How It Began for Me

Before we get too far into the details of my story, I want to provide some details relating to the disease. Then I invite you to read how it started for me. The National Multiple Sclerosis Society's Web site is the source of the disease facts. I have found their information easily understood.

According to the National Multiple Sclerosis Society's (NMSS) Web site,

> MS is thought to be an autoimmune disease that affects the central nervous system (CNS). The CNS consists of the brain, spinal cord, and the optic nerves. Surrounding and protecting the nerve fibers of the CNS is a fatty tissue called myelin, which helps nerve fibers conduct electrical impulses. In MS, myelin is lost in multiple areas, leaving scar tissue called sclerosis. These damaged areas are also known as plaques or lesions. Sometimes the nerve fiber itself is damaged or broken.

I like to think of myelin as the outside of a telephone cable and a MS person's body as the telephone to which the cable is connected. When that cable is damaged or broken, the phone doesn't work properly. As a result, conversations sometimes sound crackly and sometimes there is static. Crackly conversations and static may be likened to numbness and tingling in a MS person's legs.

According to the NMSS Web site:

> Symptoms of MS are unpredictable and vary from person to person and from time to time in the same person. For example, one person may experience abnormal fatigue, while another may have severe vision problems. A person with MS could have loss of balance and muscle coordination, making walking difficult; another person with MS could have slurred speech, tremors, stiffness, and bladder problems. While some symptoms will come and go over the course of the disease, others may be more lasting.

The NMSS Web site lists the following symptoms:

> Bladder dysfunction, bowel dysfunction, changes in cognitive function, dizziness and vertigo, depression and other emotional changes, fatigue, difficulty in walking, numbness, pain, sexual dysfunction, spasticity, vision problems.

As stated on the Web site, not everyone gets every symptom. And, not every symptom stays around permanently. A flare-up (also known as exacerbation or an attack) occurs when the symptoms of the disease worsen. The flare-up is over when the symptoms completely go away or partially abate. This is known as remission.

What causes MS? According to the NMSS Web site:

> While the exact cause of MS is unknown, most researchers believe that the damage to the myelin results from an abnormal response by the body's immune system. Normally, the immune system defends the body against foreign invaders, such as viruses or bacteria. In autoimmune diseases, the body attacks its own tissue. It is believed that MS is an autoimmune disease. In the case of MS, myelin is attacked.

Who gets MS? According to the NMSS Web site:

> … people are diagnosed between the ages of twenty and fifty; more women than men have MS, genetic factors seems to make certain individuals more susceptible than others, but there is no evidence that MS

is directly inherited. Approximately 400,000 Americans acknowledge having MS. Worldwide, MS may affect 2.5 million individuals.

How is an MS diagnosis made? Magnetic Resonance Imaging (MRI) is a very sensitive diagnostic imagining tool. It often provides the information for the definitive diagnosis of MS. MRI scans may reveal areas of the brain that have lost myelin. A MRI may also show areas of active or recent myelin activity. A person may have a spinal tap, where the spinal fluid of a person with MS may have specific characteristics, indicative of the disease.

My initial disease symptoms were vision issues—my field of vision had big blank or empty spaces. I had bladder issues—which included urgent and frequent trips to the bathroom. I had tingling and numbness. It became really bothersome when the numbness started in my legs and feet. I found that walking became difficult. I lost my balance quite a bit and the little bit of coordination I had pre-MS, became non-existent after MS.

As the disease has progressed, my vision issues became worse. I developed a condition called diplopia. It causes double vision.

I began to find that when I stooped down to pick something up from the floor, I had to literally push myself up from the floor to stand up.

My dexterity began to be affected. For example, sometimes I needed help to put on earrings, necklaces and especially bracelets. Vertigo started to be a problem. I suffered bouts of depression. Spasticity (I call it rubber band legs) was sometimes a problem. I was very often fatigued.

The progression did not happen all at once, but I would estimate that I experienced the above build up of symptoms over the course of five years. At this stage of my illness, I deal with many, if not most of those symptoms, on a daily basis. I am fortunate that my symptoms do not include pain that some people with MS suffer, nor do I have tremors.

When I have a flare-up, I am prescribed medication in the form of steroids, including oral prednisone (pills) and solumedrol, which is given intravenously for three to five days. Steroids do not permanently fix or ease the progression of MS; they ease the inflammation and therefore, the symptoms. I consider them as medication to literally get me on my feet again.

Unfortunately, I am sensitive to the steroids. I have learned that whenever I go on a course of steroids, I also get some type of stomach aid (I call prednisone my "gut buster") and sleeping pills, as sleep is very hard for me to come by while taking the medications. I have learned how to adjust my diet during a medication course. For example, I keep lots of yogurt on hand to settle my stomach. I avoid sugar, as I find it adds to my revved up state. I learned that a nice cup of tea (caffeine free) takes away the metallic taste in my mouth while the IV bag is dripping. The tea is relaxing, too. I have learned that it takes my body a few weeks after all the medications have been taken for the side effects to subside.

During one of my early exacerbations, my husband, Steve took me to the emergency room because we were convinced I was having a heart attack. It was a little embarrassing, but quite a relief, to learn that it was indigestion, caused by the steroids, and not a heart issue.

I have found that my head is "fuzzy" when I am on a course of steroids. I have learned to keep my activity to a minimum, get as much rest and relaxation as possible. Besides, I really don't feel like doing much. I try very hard to communicate with my caregiver and doctors. I watch a lot of television, spend a lot of time on the couch and try not to make any life-altering decisions during that time.

When I have an exacerbation, it is difficult for me to forget the nasty side effects and start the steroid therapy. The primary reason that I avoid making a phone call to my neurologist's office is because the steroids are not kind to my body. It's tough to remember that they are typically extremely effective for me. It's tough for me to admit this, but part of me resists, what I consider, "surrendering" myself to the disease. However, when I think of leaping buildings in a small bound or any of the other paybacks, I get the courage to make the call. Not all MS persons react as strongly to the steroids as I do. I hope you fall into that category. But if you don't, just remember, you really feel better afterwards and the therapy is worth it.

3

Doctor, Doctor, Give Me Some News

Most of us with multiple sclerosis are actually relieved when we get the diagnosis. This is due to the fact that we have known for months—and sometimes even years—that something was wrong.

As discussed previously, my problems first manifested in the form of eye issues and bladder problems. I also became tired quite easily, and I was intermittently numb in a few places. I saw various doctors for each of these different issues. I went from doctor to doctor to doctor, but my problems remained a very frustrating mystery. I knew something was wrong. I felt like a high-maintenance, paranoid, hypochondriac.

The first time that my symptoms got quite severe was during of a very stressful work project with a deadline that could not be missed. I noticed that I couldn't see very well out of my right eye. I blew it off and blamed it on the stress of the project, because I really didn't have time to deal with it. People with MS are usually aware that stress, lack of sleep, and heat do not help with our condition. The project packed all of them.

At the time, I was a Telecommunications Administrator. I used to say: "I enjoy Telecommunications because it's the perfect blend of technology and people, my two favorite things." The primary focus of my job was to connect the proper kind of phone equipment to fellow employee's needs. For example, when the Order Department's volume increased, it was my job to recommend and install the most appropriate phone equipment for the order takers. It was my job to keep the customers happy *and* to keep the order takers' jobs simple. In addition to telephone equipment, I also dealt with what we all came to know as "the phone company". I was responsible for making sure we didn't pay them too much! I also took care of providing cell phones for employees, long before everybody had one.

When I had my first major exacerbation, I was working on the installation of a large phone and voice mail system. It took place during the hot summer months. It included many twelve-plus-hour days, with tremendous pressure and stress. My team, vendors and I were working with a very tight budget and a very strict time frame.

I got through the project, and then I finally paid attention to my eyes. I saw my regular optometrist, who referred me to an ophthalmologist, who ordered my first round of MRIs. I then saw a retina specialist. I remember that when he had completed his exam, he gently placed his hand on mine and asked me whether I was under any stress. "Yeah, I sure am!" I told him. Then I asked him "What the heck is wrong with me?" I then visited a very prestigious eye hospital in Philadelphia and had a myriad of tests. When all was said and done, they pronounced my problem as "optic neuritis." And when my life calmed down and the weather got cooler, the problem went away—or so I thought.

After about two years, I started to have balance and walking problems. My bladder problems began again. I also had numbness and tingling in my legs and feet. As ridiculous as it sounds, these symptoms were good, in that I was finally referred to the correct specialist: a neurologist.

The neurologist listened to my story and immediately ordered copies of the old MRIs (remember the ones I had when my eye issues initially occurred?). He then ordered a new set of MRIs and a spinal tap.

The days between the MRIs, the spinal tap, and doctor visits were horrible. I was told that the cause of my issues might be lupus, Lyme disease, or multiple sclerosis.

After all the tests, the neurologist was able to make the diagnosis. I heard those words: "You have MS." Initially, I was relieved—at least there was a reason for all the medical problems; I wasn't crazy or a hypochondriac! However, this relief was quickly replaced with: "Oh my, what now? Why me?" That's when I started down my path of denial.

Many people with MS and other chronic illnesses have a similar reaction. I think my initial denial was helpful in that in enabled me to act, rather than get stuck in feeling sorry for myself.

I am lucky to have the *relapse-remitting* type of multiple sclerosis. I say "lucky," because there are other, more severe types called *secondary progressive* and *progressive* multiple sclerosis.

According to Fraser, Kraft, Ehde and Johnson in *The MS Workbook: living fully with multiple sclerosis (2006)*, relapse-remitting multiple sclerosis (RRMS) is the most common type. Persons with RRMS have sporadic flare-ups, at an average rate of about one every seventeen months, followed by a time period of neurological stability.

As reported by Fraser, et al., about two-thirds of the persons with RRMS progress to secondary progressive MS (SPMS). People with SPMS have a gradual, progressive decline. The course of the illness continues; there is no remission of the disease.

Another type of MS is called primary-progressive MS. Fraser, et al. tells us that patients with PPMS begin with progressive course of the illness; they do not have periods of relapse.

I would venture a guess that when anyone's own diagnosis of MS was made, and it became public knowledge, many of their friends and family told them about someone they knew who had MS. And most of those people, I'm sure were told, were living quite happily. I heard numerous testimonies such as these and I found it comforting to find out that so many people were living fairly well with the illness—but that still didn't really make it any better. I even found out that a lot of famous people have MS: they include Annette Funicello, Montel Williams, Teri Garr, country-and-western singer Clay Walker, and David Lander (Squiggy from *Laverne & Shirley)*, just to name a few.

4

Testing, Testing, 1, 2, 3 …

If you have multiple sclerosis, your diagnosis probably included MRI testing. As part of living with MS, your doctor will order MRIs periodically, in order to check on the disease. An MRI (magnetic resonance imaging) is a test that allows your doctor to see inside your body without surgery. It does this by using a big magnet and computer technology to take pictures.

Your neurologist may order different types of MRIs. My doctor usually orders pictures of my brain, spine, and thoracic, with contrast. Contrast, or gadolinium, is a dye that helps the doctors to see certain areas of the pictures better.

The tests last from twenty-five to forty-five minutes each. They do not hurt in any way, but they *are* extremely uncomfortable. You lie on a small, narrow bed, which is located directly in front of a big round opening (it reminds me of a tunnel entrance). The technician usually gives you earplugs and places a pillow under your knees to make it as comfortable as possible. Once you are all set up, the technician slides you into the big round opening, which is actually a huge magnet, or what I call "the tube." The tests require you to stay completely still. Every time I have a scan, my nose itches the minute they slide me into the tube. I always dress comfortably; I wear two pairs of socks and a sweater, as the room is usually freezing cold. The technician tucks a blanket around me, which keeps me warm and also helps me to stay still.

When getting an MRI, you cannot have any metal at all on your body. I leave all my jewelry at home and wear a sports bra to avoid metal hooks. If you forget and have something metal on your body, there are usually lockers available for you to store your personal items.

Speaking of clothes, a common worry is, "Will I have to take my clothes off?" In my experience, I have been able to leave all of my clothes on for most of the scans. There *is* one type of scan that requires you to take your clothes off, except for your underpants. The facility that usually does my testing provides pajama-like pants and a top, which make the procedure more comfortable.

If you are claustrophobic, be aware that there are "open" MRI facilities. I have never had that type, but I understand that they make all the difference for someone who just can't stay in the tube. Some people receive medication that relaxes them. I also know that there are facilities that offer headsets and music to their clients. The music is a great distraction, and it also masks the noise from the machine.

Once you are in the tube, the technician speaks to you throughout the testing. I find it very reassuring to hear her voice. The test consists of a series of segments of time, accompanied by various loud banging sounds. The loud knocking noises are different for each segment: one type sounds like a jackhammer; another, a drill; and yet another, a mixer. The noises include both high-pitched and low-pitched sounds. Before each test segment, the technician tells you how long it will last; for example, he or she says "This one will be three minutes long." It helps me get through each series a little easier, because I know what to expect. I usually pass the time with prayer, or sometimes I count.

Yes, the noise is terrifying for the first few times, but you get used to it. In fact, it actually becomes *lulling* after awhile. Believe it or not, during my last scan, I dozed off! Not for very long, mind you, but I napped for a minute or two. I hope I didn't snore.

If your MRI includes contrast, you can expect that close to the end of the testing, the technician will slide you out of the tube and inject dye into your arm via a needle. I don't mind the injection, because that means the testing is almost over! After the contrast has been injected, the technician slides you back into the tube and takes a few more pictures. And then, thankfully, you are done.

In recent times, as my MS has been active, my neurologist has ordered MRIs every two years. Most of my friends with MS follow that same schedule. And while I don't particularly enjoy them, I know it's a very good status check on my disease. I believe the best way to get through MRIs is to find out what works for *you*. Perhaps some of the tips I have mentioned may help.

5

The Office

At the time of my MS diagnosis, I was working as a Telecommunications Administrator at a wonderful local company. It was (and still is) fondly referred to as "the Tile". The company had a very good reputation, and was known as being an excellent employer.

My mother had been an employee at the Tile for several years, and I had listened to many years of dinner-table stories about the people and the place. When I graduated from high school, it was only natural for me to work there, also. I felt like I knew all of the people, and it also made it much more convenient to drive my mom back and forth to work each day, as she didn't drive. I had college aspirations, but just didn't want to tackle school full time. The Tile promoted from within and encouraged employees to improve their skills and gain education through their tuition assistance program. I took advantage of the program and received a degree taking evening classes at a local college, with the company's assistance.

In return, I remained a very loyal employee. I was fortunate to be promoted to various continuingly-responsible positions as my knowledge and experience increased. I was fortunate to be at the right place, at the right time and became quite interested in Telecommunications when the field was quite new. I was very proud of being a "woman in a man's world". Back then, most Telecommunications jobs were typically held by men.

When I was diagnosed with MS, I had worked at the Tile for seventeen years. The people I worked with were like family. Most of my associates knew of my diagnosis immediately. It was very touching to know that so many people cared as they expressed their concern via cards, flowers, and telephone calls. Their support was quite special to me.

After my diagnosis, I received treatment to reduce the inflammation and arrest the exacerbation. Thankfully, I was able to receive the medication totally at home, which made me quite happy. The hospital was the last place I wanted to be. A visiting nurse came to our home and inserted a catheter into my arm. She then started an intravenous drip of solumedrol, which is a strong steroid. The dosage was a one hour infusion per day for seven days. The nurse visited a few times during that time, she took blood, and checked on my general condition. My future husband, Steve, took a very active role in the therapy. He hooked up the IV bag many of those seven days. His involvement in the therapy went a long way to make it easier for me. As suggested by the nurse, we recruited a backup. We were fortunate that Steve's mother was able to do the job. After the seven days of solumedrol, I was prescribed oral prednisone (another steroid) for a week. I started out with three pills per day and tapered off as the week continued. It is very important that a person taking steroids, especially in the quantities described, not stop in the middle of a course of treatment. And, believe me, there were many days when I wanted to stop taking the medication, due to my discomfort with steroids.

The therapy worked very well. I felt like I could leap tall buildings in a single bound. My legs worked better. I could see much more clearly. I had more energy.

I was out of the office for about six weeks, as it was a severe exacerbation. But, as uncomfortable as the treatment was, it certainly was effective.

I was at ease with the fact that my co-workers knew of my illness. I did not feel that they treated me any differently as a result of knowing my condition. When I returned to work, many of my co-workers were quite helpful in assisting my movement in the office, understanding my need to have frequent bathroom breaks, and expressing genuine concern for my well-being.

Unfortunately, the Tile was sold. It was a very sad time. I had to say goodbye to many people who had been an important part of my life from both a personal and professional perspective. I began working at another local company. The new job was quite appealing because I was working in a very warm and cozy environment. It was just what I needed upon leaving the Tile. I was upfront about my medical condition to my new employer, in spite of many people's recommendations against doing so. Legally, I was not required to share my medical condition. But, I wanted to be completely honest with them.

I was quite happy to find out that my new employer was accepting and understanding of my MS. I did not make it general public knowledge, but when necessary (when I was having difficulty walking), I shared the information with the appropriate persons. I was not treated negatively as a result of people knowing about my illness.

I continued to work in Telecommunications, as a Manager. Just like the Tile, it was at a manufacturing plant, but on a much smaller scale. My job duties were similar to what I had previously done. I managed the company's phone and voice mail systems. I was the liaison to all telecom vendors (including long distance, pagers, cell companies and wire guys). I was responsible for telecom functionality at all company locations.

I refer to my second employer as "my in-between job." It was a family-owned business and the perfect place to go and heal after working through the nightmare of the Tile being sold. After doing the job for two years, I felt that I needed something more challenging. I enjoyed learning new things and project managing multiple tasks. Due to the size of the in-between company, such opportunities did not exist.

I found my next and most recent job to be extremely challenging. I accepted a position with a very large company, which paid considerably more money. A former co-worker and friend recruited me and knew I had MS. I did not feel the need to share any further.

I loved what I did in my corporate job. I learned a lot and met some incredible people. Unfortunately, the job was brutal for my MS. I worked long hours. I traveled quite a bit during the first few years. The commute was a bear. It was tremendously stressful. Very few people knew of my condition.

Then, I began having obvious problems. I fell a few times. I began having severe vertigo and needed to be driven home a few times. I looked like hell. I was tired all the time. I think I had four exacerbations during my six years with them. And, the remissions didn't feel like remissions! I began to feel so rotten it was difficult to continue to do my job to my personal satis-faction. I was fortunate that when my condition became known to my fel-low workers, they were quite supportive.

I was very lucky to have had three very good jobs during my working years. Not only did I love what I did, but I was able to work with very spe-cial people. Did people treat me differently because of my MS? Fortu-nately, no, they did not.

6

Getting—and Staying—MS Smart

I am a control freak. I like to know all the details about *how* to fix something and facilitate getting it done. I approached MS in the same way. I wanted to know how it could be "fixed" and what I needed to do to fix it. Guess what? I learned that there *is* no cure. I decided that I needed to do whatever I could to prepare myself for the cure, when it does end up being discovered. I did not—and still don't—want to regress to a point that will be beyond repair when the cure comes, so I learned how to get and stay smart about MS in a number of ways.

You can visit your doctor a few times a year and hope that you get the latest and greatest updates from there. But because I am a very impatient person, that isn't enough for me, so I regularly surf the internet, read books, listen to teleconferences, and connect with the National Multiple Sclerosis Society. The society is a veritable font of valuable information. I network with other people with MS and their families to hear what treatments they are receiving and how MS affects them. I attend the MS conference each year, where I can hear about the latest research and what's coming down the pipeline. It's a wonderful opportunity to talk to people, like me, who have MS.

There are many local support groups for persons with MS and other chronic illnesses. You may have to try out a few different groups and/or meetings, as not all meetings work for all people. They can be intimidating because you may meet people who are farther into the course of the illness than you are. But, the groups can be a great source of moral support, information and a place to communicate with others who understand.

You will undoubtedly have help keeping up-to-date on the latest news about MS. I am fortunate because when there is something new about MS in the press, on line or on television, I generally hear about it from others, such as loved ones. I find such contact very touching.

A few years ago, I was fortunate to meet some very special people with MS at an MS aquatics class. The fact that they went to the trouble of getting to the pool twice a week showed me that they did not feel sorry for themselves. We commiserated and shared our experiences with each other in a very positive way.

I found that drug companies that manufacture MS drugs have good Web sites, and other forms of communication, to keep people informed of their offerings.

I have shared my favorite books and Web sites in Chapter 12, The List Chapter.

7

The ABC's

When I was first diagnosed, no medications were available to treat multiple sclerosis. I was very fortunate, though, because within a few months of my diagnosis, the first drug to treat MS, Betaseron, became available. Because so many patients wanted the drug and there were limited supplies available, the drug company held a lottery to determine who would receive the drug. I have always been thankful that it was the only lottery I have ever won. I had a good number and was able to begin treatment fairly quickly.

It is widely recognized that as soon as a person is diagnosed with MS, they should begin taking one of the MS medications. These medications may delay the progression of the disease and may even increase the chances of lessening the number of future exacerbations. You may have to try a few of the drugs until you find out which one is right for you, and I think you will be glad you did.

When I began taking Betaseron, the injection process was complicated: it required a series of steps to get the drug ready to be injected. The last step was the one that I minded the most. I had to place the medication vial between my palms and roll the vial back and forth, in order to ensure that the medication was properly mixed and ready to be injected. This step took ten minutes. I was always very anxious to just get the whole thing over with. Betaseron is taken every other day, in the evening. The next day, I usually complained profusely about the process to my good friend and co-worker, Mark.

Well, my complaining was not going unheard. At Christmas time that year, I opened one of the most special presents I have ever received—Mark had fashioned a machine to do the mixing for me! It was a fascinating invention. He had used an electric pencil sharpener, a wooden spoon, and he had placed foam inside a camera-film case to create the mixer. It was fabulous! At mixing time, I simply had to pop the vial into the film case and turn the mixer on. It wasn't very pretty, and it was very noisy, but it did the job. I think of the mixer very fondly and its inventor even more so.

That mixer was very well-used—so well-used, in fact, that I soon grew concerned that I would have to go back to manual twirling. And then, one night, the mixer ceased functioning! Not to worry, though, as my husband, Steve, seized the opportunity to play with toys. The next Saturday he went shopping. Very soon after he got home, the entire living-room floor was covered with pieces from an Erector set. My husband created a mixer with the Erector set and a battery pack. We affectionately called it R2D2, and it worked quite well as a mixer for a long time.

After Betaseron, a couple of new MS drugs, Avonex and Copaxone, became available. These three drugs cleverly became known as "the ABC drugs," because of the first letter of each drug's name (Avonex, Betaseon and Copaxone). Within a few years, a fourth drug, Rebif, also became available. More recently, Novantrone and Tysabri have become available for MS patients.

The injection protocols for many of the MS drugs have improved, so that many of them can be delivered directly to your home, prefilled in the syringe and ready to be injected. They do not require mixing.

I have been on four of the drugs available for relapse-remitting MS. I changed medications for various reasons. I tried Avonex because it reduced my injections to once a week. When I had side effects, I tried Rebif, which is an injection, done three times per week. I did not take it for very long, as I began to have severe dizzy spells. So, I went back to Betaseron. I was quite frustrated when I had to stop taking Betaseron due to depression. I am now on Copaxone, which is a daily injection. I was hesitant to take a drug which required a daily injection, but I can honestly say that it is not a problem.

These drugs are administered via either subcutaneous or intramuscular injection. Betaseron, Copaxone and Rebif are subcutaneous injections. A needle is injected below the skin and the drug travels via the blood vessels to the blood stream. Avonex is an intramuscular injection, which uses a longer needle to reach muscles, which are deeper in the body.

You are probably wondering which injection hurts more, aren't you? Well, I have to say that the subcutaneous injections are less painful, but the drugs administered subcutaneously are taken more often. The intramuscular injection is more painful, but it only happens once a week.

I administer my current drug, Copaxone, via a neat injection device. This device makes the needle-sticking process simple and less scary. The injection device preparation process is detailed in the materials that are shipped with the device. In order to ease any trepidation you may have, let me review what I do on a daily basis. It is really quite simple and fault-proof.

I remove the prefilled syringe from the refrigerator when I pour my orange juice each morning. While I complete my morning tasks, such as making the bed, it gives the drug a few minutes to warm up. Then, I gather the materials I need to complete the injection, which includes: the needle, a cotton ball, an alcohol pad, the injection device and a sharps disposal container (I use old detergent bottles). I insert the prefilled syringe into the injector. I then select an injection spot. I usually use my abdomen, as it's the easiest place for me to reach. I swab the area with the alcohol pad; hold the injector over the spot. I then press the "firing button" on the injector and count to ten. I choose not to look. But, I can feel the injection, as well as hear the medicine being released from the device. I then remove the injector, and press a cotton ball against the site.

I clean up by removing the used syringe from the injector, and placing it in the sharps disposal bottle and throw out the alcohol pad, cotton ball and any other trash. The whole process takes about five minutes.

The injection does not really hurt. I feel a slight pinch and sometimes it bleeds a little. I have learned that if I take my shower directly following the shot, it helps take away the sting.

You can choose from several different injection locations. If someone is helping you, more areas are available. There is a lot of valuable information provided by the medication companies about injection sites. When the drugs are delivered to your home, they come with an instruction sheet.

On the sheet, there are diagrams of the potential sites. I cannot stress enough the need to rotate sites. In other words, don't inject into the same site repeatedly just because you can reach it the best or it hurts less; find a way to use different spots. I created a pattern that works quite well for me. In the beginning, I found that writing down the injection site that was used each day on the calendar helped me to keep things straight. You may find that it works for you, too. When my husband injects me, he usually injects into my hips or butt. I usually ask him to inject a few mornings each week. I inject on days that he's not awake!

Avonex, Betaseron and Rebif are all interferons, which sometimes cause flu-like symptoms. They are nightly injections, and the recipient can sleep through any rough, post-shot side effects. When I was taking an interferon, I would wait until I was ready for bed; then, I would take two acetaminophen tablets, and complete the injection. In most cases, I slept through any nasty flu-like side effects.

Copaxone is a different drug type and does not cause those types of side effects. I like that I can take it in the morning. It is out of the way for the day and I don't have to think about it again until the next day.

Yes, the injections stink, but I can honestly say that they have become a regular part of my morning routine. And, as unpleasant as the injections have been, I am extremely thankful that these drugs are available. I believe they have reduced the number of my exacerbations. I believe that they are all bridges to a cure.

8

Things They Don't Tell You About

If you know anything at all about MS, you know that there are some rather nasty things about it that make life ... ummm ... *interesting*. If you read about MS in a medical book, you will see very clinical symptoms, such as difficulty in walking, fatigue, bladder dysfunction, depression, speech problems, and vertigo.

Let me translate that for you:

You stumble, trip, and fall a lot; you can't stay awake past 9:00 PM; you make frequent and urgent bathroom visits; you may see a psycho-therapist. You sometimes talk like you have been drinking. And, there are days when you can be a bit dizzy.

Now, as you can imagine, all of these items can cause someone with MS some grief. Many of us have found ways to lessen the potential discomfort of these symptoms. Let me share some of these with you. Feel free to laugh, as many of us have found that laughing is quite therapeutic.

I have difficulty walking most of the time, and I am too proud to consistently use a walking aid. In order to lessen the falling potential, I always wear flat shoes. I walk close to walls and always position myself next to a stairwell's handrail. If I am in a group, I make sure that I sit down when/if possible, and I try to position myself near a person who understands my plight and will assist me if required. When I step off a curb, I use the ramp section of the sidewalk whenever possible or seek assistance from companions.

Fatigue can be bothersome for a nosy person like me. I try to take a nap every day, and I try very hard to get at least eight hours of sleep every night. I have the best energy and yawn the least in the morning. As a result, I try to schedule appointments, commitments, and fun time for mornings. If I need to be awake for an evening function, I make sure I get forty winks prior to leaving the house and try not to have anything scheduled for the morning the next day.

I am the thirstiest person alive. When I have to go somewhere, I plan my fluid intake accordingly. I avoid caffeine and other diuretics. I avoid drinking anything after 8 PM. If I do have a beverage after that time, I make sure the bed is protected, in case of leakage.

I have had a few severe bouts of depression. I have been a frequent flyer at a therapist's office for years, which has been quite helpful.

I stopped drinking alcohol over a year ago. I was a social drinker, and I'll admit that I really liked the stuff. But, as per doctor's orders, I discontinued it when I started taking some medications that don't agree with booze. I am telling you this because I slur my speech sometimes, and slurred speech in combination with walking issues and vertigo may lead people to believe that I am drunk. And you can imagine just how bad things were when I *did* drink. As a result of my lack of drinking, I have found that I slur and stumble less at parties. I also enjoy being the most sober one there and find it as amusing as, and sometimes funnier than, before—and without the headache the next day. The part that I now enjoy the most is watching my friends singing karaoke *without* a karaoke machine, with the knowledge that I will be laughing about it more than *they* will, the next day.

I am a very structured and organized person. This quality has been quite helpful, as I have found that the more planning I do, the easier things are to anticipate and enjoy. If I am going somewhere new, I have angst about the destination, such as: *Will there be steps? I hope there are railings. I hope we don't have to walk too far once we get there. Will there be places to sit down? Are the bathrooms convenient?* I suggest that you learn as much about your destination as possible before you go, and try to go places with people who understand your condition. You will enjoy everything so much more.

I accompanied a friend to a wedding, and the location was a few hours away, which necessitated an overnight stay. My friend was quite aware of my needs, so travel was fine. When we got there, we found that the hotel was MS-friendly; having both a ramp and an elevator, and our hotel-room bathtub had handrails. The wedding was to be held at a church that was a distance from the hotel, and we had no idea of the church layout. Luckily, we went to the rehearsal the night before the ceremony. My dear friend, knowing I needed the information, asked the priest where the bathroom was located. To our horror, it was located behind the altar—it is obvious to me that the architect did not know anyone with a bladder problem. It was necessary to walk onto the altar (steps and no handrails) and open a door to the area in which the restroom was located, right behind where the bride and groom would be saying "I do." Immediately, all I could picture was a two-hour ceremony and me needing to use the bathroom numerous times throughout; I envisioned myself falling on my way to the altar—all in front of a packed church! In the end, because of these considerations, I opted not to attend the ceremony. See? It's all about planning.

I must admit that I am much steadier on my feet when I use a walking aid. I can't stress to you enough to use one when necessary. I have three different canes: a pretty one, a convenient one and a sturdy one. There are some good choices out there. I purchased the pretty cane, as I figured that if I had to use one, it had to be stylish. I bought it on the Internet. I later learned that one of my fellow MS friends sells canes that are beautifully decorated. My next cane purchase will be made from her. My convenient cane is collapsible. It is very cool and extremely handy. It's useful when I need to use a cane to get somewhere but want to put it out of sight (into my briefcase or backpack) when I get there. It was inexpensive and purchased at Wal-Mart; it is definitely something you should check out. I also own a cane with a four-legged platform on the bottom of the pole. I call it "my stage cane." Certain life situations require me to lean, and it is helpful at those times. For example, it is very difficult to walk on the beach. The stage cane is wonderful to lean on when walking on the sand. Another use for the stage cane includes formal events, when it's just not appropriate to hang on to your partner or the wall.

I have learned that dogs sometimes react to a person with a cane. They know that something is different. I think that it may even be a bit intimidating for them to look up and see a stick. If you just give the dog a moment to check you out, sniff the cane, they usually forget about it.

I typically avoid buffets, if at all possible, when I go out to eat. It is something that most folks don't even think about. I have found that it is impossible to balance a plate, using a cane. Plus, I can never manage to select the food that I really want, as it is always on the serving plate in the back.

And, now, I'll mention the one benefit of having MS that "they" don't tell you about—yes, there is one. During the holidays, when most shoppers are impatiently circling mall parking lots, all we MSers have to do is hang that blue and white handicapped tag on the mirror and pull into a parking space that is nice and close to the door. And, in all seriousness, thank goodness we can do that. If not, I don't think I would be shopping in a store at all! If you have MS but don't have a handicapped tag or a handicapped license plate, I strongly urge you to get one. With your doctor's approval on the application, it is a simple task—and *well* worth it.

9

Gotta Go, Gotta Go!

A major MS problem for me is bladder issues, which are embarrassing, to say the least. I am fortunate that most of my friends and family understand this issue and help me avoid potentially horrific situations.

I remember many situations, such as trips to shopping malls, business meetings, drives in cars, rides in airplanes, which included some discomfort, accidents, and/or pit stops. One time, I was on my way to a shopping-outlet complex with a friend. It was a long drive, and I had "one of those times." It turned out to be a very convenient destination, because, upon arrival at our shopping destination, I was able to purchase and put on a dry pair of pants to get me through the rest of the day (thank goodness!). Since then, I have learned to schedule my fluid intake better. Sometimes that helps, but sometimes, it doesn't make a bit of difference. MS is so unpredictable. I am always prepared for the worst: I now carry a pair of panties in my purse.

I have learned that whenever the opportunity presents itself, you should use the restroom—you may regret it later if you don't. I have learned that it's better to excuse yourself from a conversation, meeting, church service, or movie, than to have an embarrassing accident. My husband is convinced that we have stopped in every restroom on the East Coast! One time, out of complete desperation, I stopped at a baseball field and used a port-a-potty!

I have also learned that anyone with bladder issues should see an urologist. It's a slightly demoralizing experience, due to the fact that you actually have to admit out loud that you have leakage problems. But, I am glad that I did it. I was prescribed oxybutynin, which is used to relieve urinary and bladder difficulties, including frequent urination and the inability to control urination. The medication has decreased some of my issues—and every little bit helps.

Last, but not least, I have found a company, HDIS, that sells all kinds of personal-protection items. I have included their contact information in The List Chapter of this book. They have a wonderful catalog that details the products they have available. Since personal-protection products are the only things they sell, you don't have to be embarrassed to talk to them; they have heard it all. And, most importantly, you can have your monthly supply of products delivered to your home in a plain, brown box. No more grocery-store purchases that cause the adolescent bagger to turn bright red when packing your bags!

10

The Perfect Fit

I was diagnosed with multiple sclerosis in June of 1993, and I was married in September 1993. Please note that the wedding came *after* the diagnosis. Yes, he married me anyway. As a very good friend of mine put it, "Most men would have walked." My man did not.

Before I knew I had MS, Steve and I met. We were in our thirties; both of us had bad relationships behind us; neither of us was really looking for love. I don't want to sound trite, but it confirmed to me that "it" happens when you aren't looking. And, boy, did it knock both of us on our butts! We were crazily in love; we both clicked so well that it was scary. I beamed constantly. I remember thinking that my life was finally turning out the way I had dreamed it would. Until …

For a few years prior, I'd had various, seemingly unrelated health issues. In June of 1993, however, I began to have major issues. That was when it finally got put together and I heard "You have MS." My future husband was with me every step of the way, talking to me while I was in the MRI tube and pushing me in a wheelchair to the spinal tap (and I still have not forgiven that hospital volunteer for flirting with him that day!). We talked about not going through with the marriage because of the complications of my condition. I was fearful that I was burdening him with future full of questions and pain. I wanted him to be happy. I remember a conversation during which he said, "I have thought about it, and I want to marry you." I have never felt more loved than at that moment in my life.

I was put on a course of steroids, which got me back on my feet, and we were married three months after the diagnosis. When I describe our wedding to people who were not there, I always tell them that there was not a dry eye in the house during the vows—especially during the "in sickness and in health" part. I have been told by people that it was the best wedding that they have ever been to. People have commented on the way that my husband and I looked at each other.

Following the wedding, a dilemma was "To be, or not to be parents." It was a very big question for us. We had been told by the doctors that it was possible for us to have kids, but our research indicated that, although MS mothers-to-be usually felt great during the pregnancy, after the arrival of the baby, an exacerbation usually occurred. We ultimately decided that children would not be a good choice for us. We felt that it would not be fair to anyone involved: not to Steve, not to me, and, *especially*, not a child. We still believe we made the right choice. I must say, though, that there are times when we wonder what it would have been like. We always tell our nieces and nephews that they will need to take care of us in our old age, since we don't have kids of our own to do it!

When I found out that MS medications are taken via injection, I was more than freaked out at the idea of sticking a needle into my own body. Steve did most of my injections for a long time. I would prep the drug, swab the area with an alcohol pad, hold the needle above the injection site, and then chicken out! I just couldn't do it. But there he was, ready to bail me out every time. Steve was always dreaming up ways to make it a more comfortable experience. He would crack jokes, tell me about his day, or remind me of a really pleasant time we'd had together, such as a vacation. We even got into the habit of singing songs during the process!

Since the whole injection process has improved dramatically, I now do most of the injections myself. I am quite proud of the fact that I have finally conquered my fear, and it is very empowering to do them myself. There are still certain areas that I ask Steve to do, though, because they are hard for me to reach. I am thankful that my husband was so good about it until I was ready for it. He often told me that it hurt him more than it hurt me. Because we share in the injection responsibility, it is one of the ways in which we face the disease together—and that means a lot.

In some cases, MS can have a negative effect on a person's sex life. I have very little to say on this subject, except that my husband and I have found that MS has been a catalyst to bring us even closer together. That intimacy extends into all areas of our lives, including sex. So, yes, MS has affected our sex life—but most certainly not in a bad way.

I have learned that one of the hardest ways of living well with MS is accepting that I can't do some household things. For example, I can't weed the gardens when they need weeding. I can't drag the trash can down the driveway on trash days. I can't shovel snow in the winter. To compound the helplessness of it all, I am quite impatient. When I see that a chore needs to be done, I want it done right away. Steve, on the other hand, takes a much more relaxed approach to the state of the house. For reasons that are sometimes impossible for me to understand, he doesn't have the same sense of urgency that I do. Over time, thank goodness, I have learned that the tasks happen eventually, and even if they don't, it's not a big deal. I am fortunate that Steve doesn't consider my impatience a big deal. He has taught me a lot about not sweating the small stuff. He has also taught me a lot about humility.

I love Steve, even when he says stuff like "Weebles wobble, but they don't fall down." He makes me laugh. He has supported me and *continues* to support me through difficult physical and emotional times, as I am working hard to take better care of myself. As one wise person said to me, while I was bemoaning the horrors that I was going through and how tough it was on our marriage, "When you do things to help yourself feel better, all of your relationships will feel better, too." I believe our marriage is stronger now than ever. It's just like my husband said when we were first married: the early years were the easy ones, and the hard work comes later. I am so lucky that we are the perfect fit.

We know by now that I fall on occasion. I have learned the tuck-and-roll routine, and I typically get up unscathed. We were vacationing at the Jersey shore and, while entering an ice cream parlor, I tripped and had a rather nasty fall. Steve assisted me in getting up and out of the store in quick measure. I was more mortified than anything else. He got me to a bench outside and we sat there while I recovered. When I was calmed down, he turned to me and said, "Why didn't you stay on the floor? After winning the lawsuit, we could have bought that shore house we want." I laughed and forgot about my bruises. *That's* why I love him.

11

And This One Is Juuuuust Right

When I think about the many houses that my husband and I have lived in, I am reminded of that kids' story that I have always loved, *Goldilocks and The Three Bears*. Steve and I have been together for fifteen years and have lived in four different houses, plus a temporary stay at my in-laws.

Buying and selling houses makes for lots of stress, physical activity, planning, and angst. Many of our friends and families claim to have run out of "S" pages in their address books due to the number of times our information changed.

House Number One was a small, two bedroom townhouse. I had bought it before I knew Steve. My brother joked that I found him in the basement when I moved in, as our relationship started at the same time as the address change. We lived there for about five years. We were happy with the house, although it was quite small and our belongings were overflowing when we moved to a single home.

House Number Two was a nice, little ranch. We had grand plans for the place. It was in a great neighborhood, but there were changes we wanted to make. We decided to sell it when the costs to complete the remodeling were estimated to exceed the value of the house.

House Number Three was quite large, a contemporary ski-lodge-like house, the likes of which we thought we never would own; and when we finally had the chance, we went for it! We called it The Chateau. Both Steve and I were thrilled to entertain in a house with a huge kitchen and plenty of room for guests. It was located on a nice wooded lot and backed up to a stream. Steve was thrilled, as often when he looked out of his home office window, he saw deer. However, when we bought the place, there was a minor detail that both of us decided to overlook. The house had steps everywhere! Psssst! I have MS and had no business living in such a house. We lasted there three years. It became too difficult for me to drag laundry up and down steps. It was tough, and sometimes impossible, for me to get the groceries out of my car and up the steps from the garage into the house. There were many days when I had a hard time stepping down the three steps into our favorite room.

As difficult as it was to leave the big, beautiful house, Steve and I agreed to find a place that would better suit my needs. It was a very difficult decision and I felt like I was robbing Steve of his dream home. But, it had gotten to the point that he was worried constantly that I would fall when he wasn't home. We sold the house.

We are now in House Number Four, which we fondly refer to as the Forever Home, as neither of us has any intention of moving again. It is a nice, small ranch. It is half the size of the previous location. It's a cozy, three bedroom home. Steve knew we had found the right place to buy when he saw the wood burning stove and the wet bar. Here's where *The Three Bears* fits in: this one is juuuuust right.

Well, almost—I fell down the only flight of steps in the house within one month of living in the Forever Home. Okay, it was not a good thing that the washer and dryer were downstairs in the basement, but those steps actually changed my life completely. It was the biggest wake-up call that I have ever had. I had some minor injuries as a result, but, most importantly, the fall was a catalyst to slow me down. It was the first thing that caused me to take a hard look at my illness and begin to accept it, listen to my body, and the professionals, and begin living well with MS.

And, by the way, we now have our washer and dryer on the main level of the house. No more express trips down the steps!

12

The List Chapter

I am a list person. I have numerous To Do lists, depending on the subject. I have grocery lists, shopping lists, Honey Do lists and Life Lists, just to name a few. I have lists of things to discuss at upcoming doctor appointments, and lists of things I would do if I won the lottery. My husband and I compare our wish lists.

Accordingly, I am sharing a few lists that include ways that I have found to make it easier for me to live well with MS.

Some of my favorite Web sites for MS information:

- Avonex: www.avonex.com

- Betaseron: www.betaseron.com www.mspathways.com

- Copaxone: www.copaxone.com www.sharedsolutions.com

- MS Awareness Foundation: www.msawareness.org

- My Website: www.livewellwithms.com

- National Multiple Sclerosis Society: www.nationalmssociety.org

- North American Research Committee on Multiple Sclerosis: www. narcoms.org

- Novantrone: www.novantrone.com

- Rebif: www.mslifelines.com

- The Montel Williams MS Foundation: www.montelms.org

• Tysabri: www.tysabri.com

Some of my favorite books about MS:

• *The MS Workbook: Living Fully with Multiple Sclerosis.* Fraser, Robert T., PH.D; Kraft, George H., MD; Ehde, Dawn M., PH.D; Johnson, Kurt L., PH.D. Oakland, CA; New Harbinger Publications, Inc., 2006

• *Speed Bumps Flooring It Through Hollywood.* Garr, Teri, with Henriette Mantel. New York: Hudson Street Press, 2005.

• *Multiple Sclerosis Q&A Reassuring Answers to Frequently Asked Questions.* Hill, Beth Ann. New York: Avery Books, 2003.

Some of my favorite products that help me live well with MS are available from:

• HDIS—Incontinence products

www.hdis.com

Things that make it easier for me to be comfortable and safe at home:

• Putting rubber bottoms on all carpets and rugs, to prevent slippage

• Installing handrails on both sides of all steps

• Keeping night-lights all over the house, but especially in the bedroom and bathroom

• Installing a walk-in shower with a handrail and stool

• Keeping handy a grabber device to get things from the shelves in the kitchen

• Removing tripping hazards

• Keeping many portable phones around the house

• Having a big screen television for "bad-vision times"

- Hiring a cleaning person

- Keeping reading glasses in every room

- Hiring a lawn person, who mows and takes care of the garden

Other suggestions for easier MS living:

- Make more, smaller, grocery-store runs, rather than one big one

- Get help with your shopping bags and large grocery store purchases, i.e., large cases of water

- Do your gift, clothing, and just-about-anything shopping online

- Do your banking online

- Pay your bills online

- Ask for help when you need it

- Don't use a step stool—they are hazardous

- Keep one calendar with all your appointments on it

- Think low-maintenance

- Keep lists

- If you think you shouldn't do something, *don't do it!*

You deserve to be pampered! Try one of these:

- A manicure

- A pedicure

- A facial

- Reflexology

- A massage

- A tall chai latte

13

Swimming Along

At around year eleven of my multiple sclerosis, I became aware of an MS aquatics class being offered very close to the office in which I worked at the time. Upon further investigation, I talked with the instructor, who had been certified to teach such a class by the National Multiple Sclerosis Society. I began attending the class. After many months, I told the instructor that the class had changed my life—and it had, in many ways.

Classes were approximately forty-five minutes in duration. The facility cooperated with MS guidelines that indicated that the water temperature should be no more than eighty-five degrees. People with MS like cooler pool water, as heat aggravates MS symptoms. This pool's temperature was very agreeable to us.

I can still remember the feeling when I was actually able to walk a straight line in the pool, something that I had not done on land in a very long time. Along with fellow class members, I marveled at my body's ability to complete various activities in the pool that were unthinkable for me on land. The exercises were specifically aimed at improving the physical capabilities of a person with MS. The classes also did wonders for the emotional aspects of the disease.

Unfortunately, I wedged the classes into my already packed workday. Two days a week, at lunchtime, I would rush off to the pool, hurry to get changed, attend the class, reverse the process, and rush back to work. So, while I learned that aquatics were excellent for my condition, I made getting to them one my many activities in an already overwhelming lifestyle. I even joined the local pool and pushed myself into going to the pool on the weekends, before work, or whenever possible. Somewhere in my disease denial, I thought that if I water-exercised enough, it would get me better.

Well, now I know that it can genuinely help me to feel better, but it has to be part of an otherwise healthy lifestyle.

In addition to learning the physical benefits of aquatics, I had the privilege of meeting several other people with MS. We were all there because we wanted to live well with MS. The thing that struck me immediately about the group was that it was not a "pity party." We all knew that we shared a rotten, chronic illness, and we helped each other through it by laughing and having a lot of fun. Many of these folks inspired me; they rode their scooters or pushed their walkers and used their canes to get around. They were not embarrassed by any of it, and any one of us would have done anything for the others. We shared doctor stories, medical information, and medication experiences. I had never had this kind of opportunity to discuss such things with people like myself. The group now has lunch together once a month, and I am thrilled to still be able to see them all regularly.

I now spend my water time with another group of very special people at a local YMCA. It is a water-walking class aimed at seniors. When I first attended the class, they welcomed me warmly, although I am sure they were a bit curious as to why I was there, as there was an obvious age difference. I told the instructor that I was there to improve my physical condition, due to the fact that I have MS. I felt it was important for her to understand my situation, in case I had any issues. I attend these classes two times per week. I have gotten to know my fellow class members; I have shared my story with them, and they have shared theirs with me. The class has been extremely positive in that I am physically much stronger than when I began attending, plus, it has enabled me to have friendships with these people.

Recently, I had a MS flare-up and was unable to get to class for a few weeks. I was so touched upon my return. My water friends embraced me like I had been gone years. And, when I got into the water and realized just how much strength I had lost over the course of the exacerbation, they encouraged me and urged me to keep on exercising. I was completely overwhelmed when the class's instructor offered to meet with me personally and provide me with personal water training. One of my class members told me I would be "fit as a fiddle" in no time. And she was right!

14

Real Friends and Family

I am very fortunate to have very special, loyal, and giving friends and family. Through all the ups and downs created by this illness, they have been there for me.

On the very first day that I went to the neurologist and it was obvious that something big was wrong, my dear friend, Stephanie, left work and sat and cried with me in my living room all afternoon until my future husband, Steve, got home. Years later, on the day that ended up being the last time I went to work, I stopped at that same friend's place of employment and sobbed about what I was about to do. With her support and encouragement, I did what I needed to and retired from my career life.

On the day that I fell down the basement steps, I was expecting a visit from another friend, Rose. She lives in Colorado, but was visiting her parents in a nearby town. Before her expected arrival time, I decided to do a load of wash. That was when I fell down the steps. I was fortunate that when I fell, I had a portable telephone in my pocket. So, while I was on the floor, after I calmed down and got the courage to move a little, I called my husband; he was several miles away, so I knew he would take awhile to get home. I was afraid to get up, as I wasn't sure what kind of damage had been done. I used the phone to call my friend and told her not to come over, as I'd had a little "accident." Nevertheless, she was by my side on that basement floor until my husband got home from work.

I have a standing Thursday lunch date with my friend, Cathy. I have known her since we were four years old. Each week, we try out different restaurants, and I thoroughly enjoy our time together. In addition to being my lunch date, she and her husband have provided support in more ways that I can even count.

I am still quite close to my grade school and high school girlfriends. We are lucky to be able to get away together on occasion. A few years ago, we were in an airport during one of our "girls' vacations." My friends have always been very cognizant of my needs. That day, I remember seeing a lady in a wheelchair being pushed through the airport by a bunch of other women. I know my friends saw it, too. It was definitely the elephant in the room. I know that if/when my wheelchair days come, my friends would push me around the world, if necessary.

My friends are my chauffeur when I can't drive. They take me to doctor appointments, especially the ones for which I need moral support (they somehow just know that I need them). They often rearrange their busy lives to help me do things that would be impossible without their help. I cannot tell you how many shoulders I have cried on or ears that I have talked off with my issues, and, for whatever reason, my friends keep coming back for more. I love them all.

I am the youngest of five children and the only girl. My brothers and I are the products of Irish, Catholic parents. My brothers have always been protective of their little sister. I think MS has been extra frustrating to them, as there is not a darn thing they can do about it. While we don't always have outwardly affectionate relationships, I know that any one of them would do anything for me.

My brother, Jim, has come to my rescue more times than I can count. He has saved me from countless car tragedies and house issues. As we have become adults, he is the family ear I can always count on. I am fortunate that I have been very close to him, his wife, and their two sons. Our mother lived with them for a while. I visited their home quite often. I was quite close to my nephews as they were growing up and have quite an attachment to them. In many ways, they make up for the fact that I don't have my own children. That family would walk on hot coals for me.

When my eldest nephew got married, it was a very emotional time. He and his lovely bride touched me in a way that, as I write this, still makes me cry. At the reception, there were these beautiful centerpieces on each table with candles, rose petals, and tent cards that read: IN LIEU OF WED-

DING FAVORS, A DONATION HAS BEEN MADE TO THE NATIONAL MS SOCIETY. Yes, I am very lucky.

My younger nephew is very special to me in many ways, as well. He has a special knack for making me laugh when I need it most. He loves to remind me of the time that Steve was out of town and there was a bee buzzing around in my house. It freaked me out so much so that I called him. "Can you come over and kill a bee?" Within a half hour, he had escorted the bee outside. By that point in the trauma and in the years after, he has had me laughing hysterically over my panic.

Both of us adore going to the shore. On a visit to my favorite Jersey shore spot, Stone Harbor, my nephew joined me on the beach. We talked, laughed, and dolphin-watched together. When the heat became too much for me, I made my way back to the hotel. It was a rather difficult walk for me, and I know my difficulty scared him. He gave me time to get settled back at the hotel, called me, and then came to the hotel to make sure I was alright. He made sure his father knew of the incident, so that my brother would check up on me when I got home.

My husband's family is quite supportive. My parents-in-law are very special to me; my parents are both deceased, so it wonderful to have them as a big part of my life. Whenever Steve and I are MS fund-raising, his entire family is always generous. One year, my sister-in-law, who is a successful jewelry salesperson, did a jewelry show at our home, and donated her earnings to the MS Society.

Several years ago, as part of my National MS Society fundraising efforts, I started The M Team. The Team has raised several thousands of dollars due to the generosity of my family and friends. Every bit goes to the cure.

I have a friend who owns a wonderful Italian restaurant. He is extremely generous to my cause. One spring, my husband and I did a fund-raiser in our home to benefit the National MS Society. Our chef friend donated his scrumptious scallops and many other incredible hors d'oeuvres. I know his food was a major attraction for our event, and we raised a good amount of money for the society. Another fund-raiser was an art show at his restaurant, which benefited the National MS Society. He is a very special friend.

I have got to be honest with you: not everyone is as supportive as the wonderful friends and family I have just talked about. You may find that some people disagree with your lifestyle or your approach to your illness. It can be very difficult to keep your head high at those times. But, I learned that those people are in the minority.

Most importantly, I have learned to fully appreciate and enjoy the wonderful family and friends that I have and hope you can, too!

15

Two Left Feet

When I was a kid, I always wanted to roller skate on the sidewalk out in front of our row house with my friends. I had a neat pair of skates, but I was a terrible skater and spent most of the time on my butt on the pavement.

During my younger days, when my friends used to do handstands, somersaults, and other gymnastic moves, I was always their "director." Even back then, there was absolutely no way I could do any of those moves.

I loved to go to the local ice skating rink. I couldn't ice skate, but it was the place for kids to hang out. When the editor of my mother's employee news magazine was looking for volunteers for a cover photo, my mother volunteered me to have my picture taken at the local ice skating rink. Yes, there I am on the cover of the January 1969 issue of the *Tile News*, on my butt, at the local ice-skating rink. I guess she forgot, that although I liked going to the rink, I couldn't stand up on the ice skates!

Once, my future husband and I were recruited to take his nephew and niece skiing. Please note the "future" part in that sentence—I was still in the early stage of our relationship where I went along with everything. From the moment my feet were clamped into those skis, I was on my butt in the snow. I was wearing a pair of borrowed, bright pink ski pants that the boys could see every time they were beginning a new run down the slope. I imagine that their observations were hysterical. Our niece graduated to the bunny slope hours before it became apparent that I could not conquer even the very small practice hill. It was such a relief when the instructor kindly said to me, "Why don't you go get warm in the lodge?" Hallelujah!

I remember joining the bowling league in my early days at The Tile. What was I thinking? As I am sure you can imagine, I had more gutter balls than strikes. But I had fun, anyway.

I have two left feet; but at least now I have an excuse to sit on the sidelines when the volley ball net comes out at picnics. I would love to do the electric slide at weddings, but I know better and stay in my seat.

16

Heart and Sole

The emotional and mental parts of my journey to living well with MS have been quite challenging for me. There were many times when I felt like I was walking that part of the journey without any shoes on my feet, or that the soles of my shoes were worn out. The road has been quite rough.

I always thought it was *me*—that I simply couldn't emotionally handle MS and that caused my depressions. I had all kinds of reasons why I was depressed. I blamed my depression on a predisposition. I blamed it on the stress of my job. I thought that perhaps my life situation caused my depression. Maybe it was menopause?

I learned a few things that made my depression, much less depressing. I learned that depression may be the result of a rough patch of life, for example, dealing with disability due to a chronic illness. Additionally, depression can also be caused by MS itself. If the myelin that covers the nerves that transmit signals affecting your mood are damaged, it may cause depression. I also learned that many MS medications may cause depression.

I learned that interferons—medications which are used to treat MS, and which I had been taking for many years—may cause depression. So I was taking a drug that caused depression for a disease that caused depression—*and* I was menopausal. I couldn't do much about my age, but I no longer take an interferon. I have had, and I am sure I *will* have, some rough times emotionally as a result of the disease, as I am sure many others with MS do.

I won't be silly enough to tell you to "snap out of it" yourself, as I know it just isn't that easy. I am telling you from my heart, that the darkness can get lighter. Different things work for different people on the journey to find that light. I am fortunate to have excellent professionals to help me in this area, and I strongly recommend that anyone with MS or any other chronic illness look for that same level of support.

I am quite happy that I learned that my depression wasn't my fault and that I learned various ways to ease the pain caused by depression. I hope that other persons with MS and their families are able to gain that understanding, as well.

17

Go Fly a Kite

I talked earlier about my Life List. The first thing on that list was to fly a kite. I had never flown a kite before, but, I finally did it.

It happened when I was vacationing at the Jersey shore with my family. We made an event out of it. We even took pictures. We took the kite down to the beach. Sand is extremely difficult for a person with MS. It is quite hard to maintain balance on the sand's surface. Fortunately, we were flying the kite at a handicapped-accessible beach, where in addition to the ramp onto the sand, there was a wooden boardwalk *in* the sand. I could stand on a wooden plank, rather than the sand, and feel secure. Steve got the kite airborne, but, when it was up there, he handed over the strings and stood behind me so that I could lean on him, enabling me to look up at the kite without getting dizzy. It was fantastic!

Number Two on my Life List was Going Fishing. I had never been fishing. I had this picture in my head of me sitting by a pond, with a fishing rod in my hand, the sun shining on my face, enjoying nature at its finest. On a trip to the beautiful mountains in northwestern Pennsylvania, I went fishing. AND, I even caught a fish! My dear friend's father was determined to help me make it happen; and, much to our delight, it did.

For a long time, I let multiple sclerosis get in the way of doing things I wanted to do. I never said out loud, "I am not doing that, because MS limits my activities." And, I don't think I even admitted it to myself. But, I have thankfully gotten over the self-imposed limitations.. I found out that even if I can't do things the way I did them before—or the way other people do them—it *is* possible to improvise, and people will enthusiastically work with me to make it happen.

There are a lot of items on my life list that I would never have dreamed I could do. Now, I don't feel so hopeless or insecure about doing them—I know I can at least try. I know that I can ask my family and friends to help me and know that they may enjoy it as much as I do.

The next item on my list is to take a sailboat ride. I would also love to visit an Irish castle. What's on your list?

18

There's No Place Like Home

Just like Dorothy in *The Wizard of Oz*, I found out that there's no place like home; unfortunately, it took more than tapping my ruby slippers together three times to find that out. I am no longer a member of Corporate America. My life does not include a brief case, a cell phone, instant messaging, an on call list, or a pager. It's different, but I am adapting to it.

When stress, aggravation, depression, lack of sleep—and yes, MS—caused me to have severe physical issues, it became impossible for me to continue in my job. When I fell down those basement steps, it finally became real to me that I needed to stop and take care of myself. The day after the fall, I went into the office with my banged-up face and told them that I was going to be out for awhile, to get myself feeling better again. I honestly thought I would return to work in a few weeks—after all, I was indispensable. Well, weeks turned into months, and here I am. I am now officially on disability. Wow, what an adjustment for me, my husband, and everyone else in my life.

A few months after I had been home from work, I remember when it finally dawned on me that it would be physically impossible for me to do my job. I was talking with a friend and I cried more than I have ever cried about this awful disease, MS. I panicked, just thinking about it. To me, my identity was tied to my job: I don't have kids. I have worked since I was eighteen. I lived, ate, and breathed work. I met my husband through work. What kind of person would I be without my job? Would people still like me? Would *I* still like me? In addition to a nice income, my job gained me respect and allowed me to feel like I was an important person. I wanted so bad to just be "normal" again.

It is a very humbling experience for a person with a disability to come face-to-face with the fact that she cannot do something (like her job) due to her illness. I have never felt more vulnerable in my life. I have dealt with some zingers, but this one has been the most difficult life experience I have had thus far.

Fortunately, I have disability insurance that contributes to our household income. But I have not been able to shake the feeling that it will all come crashing down, and we will have financial issues. And even though everyone tells you that your first social-security application will be denied, when that denial comes in the mail, it is devastating.

My husband and I always knew this time would come, but we didn't think that it would be *this* soon. We had planned for it in many practical ways. We had no idea that the practicalities were the easiest part.

Today, "normal" is a very different thing to me. I am able to get the sleep that I need. There is time and opportunity to get regular exercise. When I am tired and can't keep doing something, I stop doing it. I have even learned how to ask for help when I know I can't do something myself. Driving is something I avoid, especially if my destination is off my beaten path or at night. When that little warning voice goes off in my head, I actually listen.

When I do something like clean the house, watch David Letterman and get up at six in the morning the next day, or sign up for a college class, my favorite line is "I guess I shouldn't have done that." My hope and prayer is that, one day, I say that a lot less.

And, yes, I do even watch some daytime television. When my husband came home from work, I would say to him, "So and so was on television today, and they said blah blah blah," and Steve would get this frightened look in his eyes. At least I wasn't eating bon bons.

After being home for a while, there is only one show that has remained on my daytime list. In fact, I even record it every day, in case I am water-walking or out of the house for an appointment: it's *The Ellen DeGeneres Show*. From the first week that I was home, she has given me something to laugh about—which is a respite from my illness. My favorite part of her show is the beginning. Her monologue is always laugh-out-loud funny and I love to watch her and her audience dance. I love to dance, but don't do much of it in public any more. But, when I am alone in my living room, watching Ellen, yes, I dance! My friend, who really loves to dance, and I have dreamed of being in Ellen's live audience. Maybe someday; after all, it *is* on my Life List.

Since I am home now, I water-walk frequently, see my doctors regularly, have lunch with friends, and take naps. I have even gone to a few matinee movies.

I have learned that cats really *do* sleep most of the day. At first, Katie and Cinnamon (our cats) liked me being home, because I let them in and out of the screened-in porch all day long. That got old after a few weeks, though, and they now have their daytime hiding places. Every now and then, I hear one of them snoring in a corner. When it's feeding time, they are quite happy that I am home and they don't have to wait till all hours for me to come home and give them dinner.

I now enjoy snow. I always had the reputation for being the first one out of the office when the first snowflake fell, because driving in the snow was traumatic for me. Ironically, there was only one sizable snowstorm during my first winter home. It was awesome to look out the window and not worry about it. I no longer agonize about the weather forecast—it is possible for me to appreciate the beauty of freshly fallen snow.

I can actually say that I have hobbies now. I have found that I love to take pictures of scenery. I enjoy printing the photos and sharing them with family and friends. I also print them and have framed many of them and have hung them in our home.

I have become a bird watcher. I sit on our back porch and watch the blue jays, cardinals, finches and woodpeckers enjoy the various feeders we have. Previously, I would never have had the patience to stay put, let alone pick up a pair of binoculars to get a better look. Now, I treasure the time.

19

And the Moral of the Story ...

When I was part of the business world, I had the opportunity to mentor associates less experienced than myself. I really enjoyed doing it. If and when something they were doing went awry, and after we did the necessary repair or cleanup work, I would usually say to my mentoree, "What was the moral of *that* story?" Most times, they wanted to throw something at me, but, in the end, we both learned something from the experience, and we both knew it.

I challenge you to figure out the moral to *your* story. And since I can't ask you to do something I haven't done, I will do the same—right here, right now.

From a very early age, I knew I wanted to work in the business world. My mother was an executive secretary and I loved to hear her talk about her day. I knew that's what I wanted to do. Directly out of high school, I entered the business world. I earned my bachelor's degree at night, while I was doing the thirty-year climb up the corporate ladder during the day. I always took great pride and pleasure in what I did; I worked in the telecom field, and it was good match for me, as it blended technology and people—my two favorite things. The climb was a respectable one, and I was making good money in a nice job at a very large corporation when I exited the business world.

So, what's the moral to my story? Well, it took me a long time to figure it out, and today, I still work on it. Here are some things that I have learned:

- Money isn't everything.

- People disappoint sometimes, and you can't take them too seriously.
- My health is more important than getting that project plan done.
- I can still contribute to the world without a BlackBerry, pager, or laptop.
- I like to dabble in some creative things, such as photography.
- Nature has beautiful surprises, every day.
- Selling stuff on the Internet is easy.
- After many years, I can still play the piano.
- It is possible to sit still.
- It is wonderful to see, smell, and hear the ocean, without a million other things on my mind.
- There is spirituality in my life that is indescribable.
- There are a few easy yoga poses that I have learned, and it feels great to do them.
- Having MS has created opportunities for me to meet very special and wonderful people who have touched my life in ways I could never have imagined.

Yes, I have a disability that limits what I can do—the hardest part of learning that fact was *accepting* that fact—but I do not have anything to prove to anyone, including myself. There are ways around those limitations. I am learning to keep on trying.

Most importantly, I have learned that all days will not be good days, and when I have one of those bad days, it's okay to stay home and watch television. It's important and necessary for me to pay attention to my body and slow down when it tells me to. It is possible for me to have an identity without a career. People like me just the same whether I go to the office every day or not. And some people even like me better because I don't!

I don't want to dismiss the fulfillment of having a career or insinuate that my working life was a bad thing. There was a lot of satisfaction, for me, in a job well-done. I enjoyed being a cheerleader wherever I worked. I had many fun times with wonderful people, some of whom remain a very big part of my life. Working was an educational and gratifying time in my life, and it's a big part of who I am today and who I will be tomorrow.

My wish for you is that you take the time to find those special things inside you. I am very glad that I stepped off the treadmill and learned some incredible things about myself—and that I continue to learn more and more each day.

20

If the Shoe Fits

I hope you enjoyed hearing about my journey, and I also hope that you read at least one thing that caused you to walk in my shoes—and that you found that the shoe fit. Hopefully, I shared something that makes it easier for you or a loved one to live well with MS.

I am still waiting to wear those black suede pumps with the three-inch heels. They sit on my desk as motivation. To me, they are even more beautiful today than when I bought them. I can't wait to wear them again. And, so that I can, I continue to live as healthy a life as possible. I hope you do, too. I have learned that life, with or without MS, is wonderful.

When the cure comes, I will wear my heels to the celebration party. I hope to see you there!

References

What is Multiple Sclerosis? Retrieved August 1, 2007, from
http://www.nationalmssociety.org/site/PageServer?pagename=
HOM_ABOUT_what_is_ms

Symptoms Retrieved August 1, 2007, from
http://www.nationalmssociety.org/site/PageServer?pagename=
HOM_ABOUT_symptoms

What Causes MS? Retrieved August 1, 2007, from
http://www.nationalmssociety.org/site/PageServer?pagename=
HOM_ABOUT_what_causes_ms

Who Gets MS? Retrieved August 1, 2007, from
http://www.nationalmssociety.org/site/PageServer?pagename=
HOM_ABOUT_who_gets_ms

Fraser, Robert T., Kraft, George H., Ehde, Dawn M. & Johnson, Kurt L.
(2006) *The MS Workbook: living fully with multiple sclerosis.* Califor-
nia: New Harbinger Publications.

978-0-595-44446-
0-595-44446-6

Breinigsville, PA USA
10 October 2010
247021BV00002B/4/A